Mona Rajeh
Shahrokh Esfandiari

A Look at Women's Professional Lives in Dentistry

Mona Rajeh
Shahrokh Esfandiari

A Look at Women's Professional Lives in Dentistry

A Qualitative Study

LAP LAMBERT Academic Publishing

Impressum / Imprint
Bibliografische Information der Deutschen Nationalbibliothek: Die Deutsche Nationalbibliothek verzeichnet diese Publikation in der Deutschen Nationalbibliografie; detaillierte bibliografische Daten sind im Internet über http://dnb.d-nb.de abrufbar.

Bibliographic information published by the Deutsche Nationalbibliothek: The Deutsche Nationalbibliothek lists this publication in the Deutsche Nationalbibliografie; detailed bibliographic data are available in the Internet at http://dnb.d-nb.de.

Coverbild / Cover image: www.ingimage.com

Verlag / Publisher:
LAP LAMBERT Academic Publishing
ist ein Imprint der / is a trademark of
OmniScriptum GmbH & Co. KG
Heinrich-Böcking-Str. 6-8, 66121 Saarbrücken, Deutschland / Germany
Email: info@lap-publishing.com

Herstellung: siehe letzte Seite /
Printed at: see last page
ISBN: 978-3-659-34680-4

DEDICATION

This thesis is dedicated to my parents for their continual support and encouragement. It is also dedicated to my loving husband and beloved children, who continue to delight and inspire me.

ACKNOWLEDGMENTS

First and foremost, all praise and heartfelt thanks are given to Allah the almighty, who gave me the strength and endurance to pursue my scientific approach. With his guidance and blessings, I successfully overcame all the challenges I faced throughout this demanding program, and successfully completed my master's degree.

I would like to gratefully and sincerely thank Dr. Richard Hovey for his guidance, understanding, and patient advice. I have been extremely lucky to have him as a supervisor. He cared very much about my work and replied to my questions and inquiries promptly. He was always approachable, and his vision and extensive knowledge of qualitative research have helped significantly in its success.

I must express my sincere gratitude to Dr. Shahrokh Esfandairi for giving me the opportunity to work on this project under his supervision. His invaluable assistance, enthusiasm, and faith have always inspired me. His goal of excellence kept me determined and focused.

I extend my sincerest thanks to my parents, Talal and Laila, who have taught me the value of hard work and education since childhood. Their continuous support and prayers brought me closer to achieving my goals. Without a doubt, I would never have become what I am today without them.

My very special thanks and love go to my husband, Fahad, for his enduring love and support. His energy, his compassion, and his belief in me are the incentives that encouraged me to continue. He always reassures me tenderly when I am under stress.

Endless love goes to my dear children, Yaseen and Haitham, for the endearing spirit they bring to my life. Seeing innocent smiles and laughter on their pretty faces has always helped me to overcome all struggles.

I am also very grateful to my sister, Mai, and my two brothers, Mohammed and Motoaz. Despite the distance between us, they were a great source of comfort and enjoyment. They always cheer me up with their high spirits and sense of humour.

I also wish to extend my gratitude to my friends for their advice and encouragement. They always listen patiently to my complaints and help me at different stages of my personal and professional life.

I would also like to thank my in-laws, Haitham and Sabah, for the care and support they expressed during my studies.

I am also extremely grateful to the Ministry of Higher Education in Saudi Arabia, which offered me a full scholarship to continue my postgraduate studies.

TABLE OF CONTENTS

LIST OF TABLES

1. INTRODUCTION

"Is there no way for men to be, but women must be half-workers"

William Shakespeare

The proportion of women in the dentistry profession has been consistently increasing over the past 40 years (1). This study explored the issues and concerns that influence professional practice for female dentists, while attempting to reconcile familial and societal pressure. Some studies have shown that gender differences influence choice of specialization, practice patterns, and professional attitudes (2, 3); while others have revealed that women favour primary care management practices, rather than other dental specialties (3). It has also been suggested that women tend to work fewer hours, work part-time, and see fewer patients than men, and are less likely to own their practices. There is also a net income discrepancy between male and female dentists (2).

Therefore, we aim to describe the issues that motivate the decisions made by female dentists, with regard to their dental practices, and to document their voices and experiences. This research also highlights some of the difficulties encountered by female dental practitioners.

Much like the author, female dental practitioners experience the dilemma of wanting to be perceived as efficient before having children, yet fulfilling their role as a mother. The driving force behind this research was the daily challenges faced in attempting to achieve professional goals, while fulfilling marital and maternal obligations. It will eventually be critical to provide a supportive workplace for female dentists in order to deliver high-quality services and to ensure that the productivity of the dental workforce is not negatively affected

2. LITERATURE REVIEW

2.1 Gender and Feminization

Recent studies examining gender heterogeneity among the health professions, and focusing on the preferential differences between men and women, have shown that many fields, including medicine and dentistry, are highly segregated by gender (4, 5); it is predominantly men that enter these professions. Unlike men, women seek jobs, such as nursing, which aid the men professions. Recent trends have found that the ongoing emergence of multiple specialties, like surgery and paediatrics, has provided women with excellent opportunities to excel in some speciality programs.

Some studies have examined the causes of the changing attitudes toward the feminization of health professions (1, 5). The contextual meaning of feminization reflects the incorporation of women into formerly male-dominated professions (1). Adams (2010) examined the nature of this feminization in healthcare professions in the United States and Canada between 1930/1931 and 2006/2008 (6). The results showed that the percentage of female practitioners employed in the health professions increased dramatically throughout this period, as many new areas of expertise emerged (6).

Reskin and Roos (1990) suggested that the increased number of women in the workforce was due to improved levels of education, social changes, and occupational changes, as well as women's increased passion with regard to practicing in the healthcare professions, along with a concomitant steady, or decreased, enthusiasm among men (7).

An additional reason for the feminization process may be the abundance of job opportunities in many healthcare sectors (8–11), and the emigration of foreign female practitioners to developed countries, such as the United States and Canada. As a result, many arguments have focused on whether the influx of women into traditionally male-dominated health occupations would lead to positive or negative consequences for dentistry (1).

2.2 Types of Dental Services Provided

Researchers have examined aspects of gender discrimination and professional equality as general issues in dentistry specialties (1, 12–14). Female health practitioners tend to enter into disciplines such as paediatric dentistry and orthodontics, which allow them to balance their work with familial obligations.

The dominance of men in high-status specialties, such as surgery, is not related to women's lack of preference for such fields, rather, this trend has occurred because of a greater number of men pursuing these specialties (15). The perception of the role of women, with regard to responsibilities, along with a significant lack of female role models in dentistry, may also be a contributing factor. Therefore, it is important to understand and foster awareness of the variables that could influence women's career choices. A second contributing factor may be that women working in traditionally male-dominated specialties may be treated differently by their male counterparts and/or superiors, colleagues, nurses, and patients while trying to demonstrate professionalism in their careers (16–18).

Recent review articles have highlighted the dramatic increase in the number of female dentists who have preferences for certain specialties in Germany, Bulgaria, and other European countries. This growth has been linked with a potential impact on the capacity of the dental labour force to provide a full range of services. There has also been a significant change in the types of treatments provided by both male and female dentists. Male dentists have predominantly chosen specialities such as periodontic, prosthodontic, and implantology, whereas female dentists have been pioneers in pedodontic, orthodontic, and dental prophylaxis (14, 17–22). This tendency was discussed by Clark et al. (2000), who generalized that women tend to be more sensitive, more altruistic, and less egotistic, and that these characteristics might be factors that contribute to their speciality choices (23). Atchison et al. (2002) addressed gender issues to compare differences in chosen practice patterns among general dentists (21). Male postgraduate dentists offered more complicated services, such as periodontal surgery, extractions, implants, and conscious sedation. In contrast, female postgraduate dentists were more willing to practice simple measures, such as space maintenance, full and partial dentures, orthodontic, and endodontic. The interim and lasting effects of postgraduate training on professional behaviours were also highlighted. The authors ascertained that gender disparity was evident in the types of services provided by postgraduate-trained dentists, and therefore there is a significant gender disparity in career patterns. However, a study conducted in Washington, D.C., by Aguila et al. (2005) did not support this assertion (2). These conflicting studies demonstrate that this issue is not well understood and is under researched.

2.3 Working Patterns (Practice Characteristics)

During the last decade, the number of dentists in Bulgaria has increased by some 24% (14); compared to the world trend of 18% (24), and the EU trend of 15% within the same period (25). Given that the number of women entering the field of dentistry increased dramatically in the 20th century (14, 26, 27), Niessen, Kleinman, and Wilson (1986) reviewed a wide range of literature on the practice characteristics of female dentists (28), and several of these studies provided evidence supporting a trend whereby women work fewer hours than men. Spencer and Lewis (1998) evaluated the discrepancy between male and female dental practitioners and observed substantial differences in working hours; females were more likely to work fewer hours than their male counterparts (29). The mean working hours per day for female dentists was 7.2, while for male dentists this figure rose to 8.1. Similarly, Brennan et al. (1992) showed that the mean hours worked per week by female dentists was significantly lower than the mean of weekly hours worked by male dentists (3). Table 1 reports the mean working hours per week among male and female dentists in several studies. Men also worked on a part-time basis less frequently than did women (22, 13, 30). Aguila et al. (2005) also noted that women see fewer patients than their male counterparts (2). The observed patterns of lifecycle labour force participation of women, and the combination of work and household responsibilities, suggest that the relationship between work status and family happiness is of importance.

Three studies addressed the issue of why women predominate in part-time work (22, 31, 32) and found that caring for children and personal choices were the most common reasons for the smaller number of weekly hours worked by female dentists. Similar research has revealed that the practicing patterns of genders differ only after the birth of a child (3, 22, 31, 33–35). These reasons all contribute to why it is important to ascertain why women in dentistry work fewer hours and why they predominantly work part-time.

In addition, some studies have revealed that the number of female dentists who take career breaks exceeds that of male dentists (3, 13, 22, 32). These studies showed that personal choice, job-hunting, personal illness, and going back to school were the main reasons for such differences. In addition, child bearing, child

5

rearing, and difficulty returning to work after vacation were issues of concern among many women.

Study	Country	Sample size Male	Sample size Female	Mean Male	Mean Female
Table 1. Working Hours Per Week: Gender Comparison					
Spencer and Lewis, 1988	Australia	657	337	8.1(hr/week)	7.2(hr/week)
Kaldenberg et al., 1995	Oregon	147	47	36.0	30.8
Newton et al., 2000	U.K.	1153	580	38.04	30.68
Adams, 2005	Ontario, Canada	350	300	39.2	35.6
Ayres et al., 2008	New Zealand	659	482	36.0	29.1

Previous studies have also indicated that, despite the increased number of female dentists in the workforce, women remain in a minority in dental academic and leadership roles, because men in the academic and private workforces have traditionally dominated these areas within the dental community. Furthermore, men with postgraduate qualifications held more senior management positions than did women, who were more likely to be involved in faculty or government positions (13, 14, 19, 21).

7

Overall, the professionalization of dental practice has resulted in the continuation and consolidation of male dominance among dental specialists. Male specialists in various fields of dentistry still far outnumber female specialists, as several studies have highlighted (1, 12–14). Table 2 summarizes the results of these studies. Despite the fact that dentistry is now becoming increasingly feminized and gender-segregated by practice setting, the hierarchies among dental professionals persist.

Table 2. Percent of Specialists: Male Vs Female				
Study	**Country**	**Sample Size**	**Specialists (%)**	
			Male	**Female**
Kaldenberg et al., 1995	Oregon	300	27.5	11.4
Katarova et al., 2004	Bulgaria	842	6	2
Adams, 2005	Ontario, Canada	800	11.5	1.5
Ayres et al., 2008	New Zealand	850	14.6	7.9

2.4 Private Dental Practice Ownership

Practice ownership trends are also linked to gender, and men are more likely to own their dental practices. Since qualifications and commitments to organizing a practice are commonly associated with men, who are considered to be the primary wage earners in their families, women tend not to own their own practices (12–14, 32). With regard to self-employment, several studies have explained the multitude of factors that contribute to a woman's choice, as opposed to that made by a man, such as differences in labour market opportunities for men and women, due to discrimination; experience and skills differentials; maternity and childcare concerns; and variations in lifetime occupational strategy (13, 36). Overall, a lower percentage of women worked in private practice compared to men (14, 29), and, in the private sector, the percentage of females working in a solo practice was lower than what was observed among their male colleagues (14, 22, 29, 37). As mentioned previously, men are traditionally and culturally considered to be the primary wage earners in their families, so male dentists have the time and inclination to develop and run a private practice. With the increase in female participation in the dental labour force, it is important to observe and evaluate the effects of gender-related distribution on dental practice.

2.6 Net Income

A gender comparison in terms of net income among dentists showed that women earn less than their male co-workers for doing the same kind of work, yet few studies have examined the differential between the wages of male and female dentists (12, 38). Aguila et al. (2005) revealed a significant difference in earnings between men and women (2); the net income of female dentists was 10% lower than that of their male counterparts. These results are consistent with those of an earlier study conducted in 1995, which found that the mean net income of female dentists was approximately $34,000 annually, while the mean net income of male dentists was approximately $68,000 annually (12). Inequities in the level of education, work experience, and working patterns may play a role in the observed differences in wage inequality.

An American Dental Association survey carried out in 1995 showed that two-thirds of female dental practitioners believed that they earned less than men. In contrast, two-thirds of male dentists believed that there was no gender disparity in dentists' earning levels (39). However, the existing data imply that the perceptions of female dentists are more accurate than those of their male counterparts.

Brown and Lazar (1998) attempted to clarify this matter by focusing on women and men who had similarities in levels of education and practice characteristics (38). The average difference in net annual income between male and female dentists was approximately $26,000, and the wage difference in hourly earnings was $12. Despite adjusting for factors such as education and practice pattern, gender was also an issue in networking, and in preferential treatment within the dental market.

Other statistical studies conducted in Canada have revealed that female dentists earn 40% less than their male peers (Statistics Canada 2008). Differences in income between men and women may occur because men prefer to own their own dental practices (clinics), unlike women, who usually work for others (1, 6, 40). The issue of men versus women income inequality is complicated and necessitates multi-level analysis that must account for ethnicity, cultural differences, and education levels. The gender wage gap may have real consequences, especially for female dentists who are also the primary earners in their families. Income inequalities undermine families' economic security (41).

2.7 Job Satisfaction

Women hold dental positions that are, on average, inferior to those held by men, and, on average, they have less autonomy, have limited opportunities for promotion, and earn less money. However, despite this, women and men have a comparable level of job satisfaction (12, 13, 42). Luzzi et al. (2005) examined differences in job satisfaction between female and male dentists, according to a variety of dimensions, such as autonomy, relationships with colleagues, relationships with patients, relationships with staff, personal time, intrinsic satisfaction, community, compensation, administrative responsibilities, and resources. The results showed that male and female practitioners varied significantly on the personal time dimension alone, which relates to satisfaction with quality and quantity of time for self and family, in that female dentists appeared to derive greater satisfaction (43). It is important to examine career satisfaction among female dentists, not only because it may improve their work-related quality of life, but also because it may improve their performance in practice.

A wide range of studies on job satisfaction and occupational stressors that affect dentists' attitudes toward their careers have been published (44–48). Two surveys were distributed to dentists in the U.S, with the aim of determining whether job satisfaction is related to certain demographic and practice characteristics (49, 50). Both of these surveys recorded lower satisfaction scores among female dentists, and, along with further analysis, revealed that the decrease in satisfaction scores was related to age and not gender. Although the dilemma of work-family conflict has become an issue of concern for most of today's female dentists, it did not have an impact on their job satisfaction.

To address these knowledge gaps, we examined the personal and professional perceptions of female dental practitioners, as well as their goals and expectations, in our study. We believe that the findings of this pilot study can lead to an improved understanding of women-related issues in dentistry and pave a path to future studies.

3. RESEARCH QUESTION/OBJECTIVE

Our primary interest was in assessing the types of barriers, if any, faced by female dentists. To further advance our knowledge, we conducted this study to understand and describe the concerns that implicitly and/or explicitly influence their practice patterns. Through this research, we hope to enhance our knowledge of evidence-based practices and to aid policy-makers on how to achieve supportive work environments and develop gender-specific incentives that meet the current professional and family needs of female dentists in Canada.

To gain insight into this topic, we employed a qualitative research approach to find answers to the following question:

- *What are the issues that influence the decisions made by female dentists, with regard to their profession?*

Study Objectives

1. Describe the factors that influence the types of practices female dentists choose to perform.

2. Lay the foundation for how female dentists perceive their profession.

4. METHODOLOGY

4.1 Research Method

The focus of the proposed research was exploratory and descriptive in nature, so we used a qualitative descriptive approach, endeavouring to learn from the participants' narratives to begin to understand their experiences (51). We also chose this method because of its suitability to the research topic, population of interest, and the data collection analysis.

Milne and Oberle (2005) applied a qualitative descriptive methodological approach to describe the self-care strategies that individuals maintain at home, and the factors that affect these individuals' decision-making processes (52). They proposed a list of questions: 1.What self-care strategies do people initiate and/or maintain in relation to their urinary incompetence? 2. What are the perceived benefits of these self-care strategies? 3. What factors influence self-care choices? 4. What factors facilitate/impede adherence to behavioural strategies? Although the content of this study was different from that of the current study, the findings and results were reported through a practical understanding of the topic, which aligned well with the intention of our research project. On the basis of the similarities between our objectives and those of Miln and Oberle, we decided that the qualitative descriptive approach was an appropriate methodology for our study (52).

Elsewhere, Sullivan-Bolyai et al. (2005) explained that the goal of qualitative description *"is not thick description (ethnography), theory development (grounded theory) or lived experience (phenomenology), interpretative meaning of an experience (hermeneutics), but, rather an accurate and relevant description of the experience depicted in easily understood language"* (53).

Sandelowski (2000) described qualitative descriptive research studies as the least theoretical among all of the qualitative approaches (54). However, the epistemological theoretical framework of our descriptive study is set within the paradigm of naturalistic inquiry (54, 55). Qualitative descriptive studies are more naturalistic in that they do not employ the theoretical underpinnings or interpretive approaches of other qualitative methodological frameworks (51, 54).

We deemed a qualitative descriptive study as appropriate for our research, as we intend to describe the reasons that affect the practice patterns of our recruited cohort of dentists, while engaged within their professional capacity, with the interpretation of data focused on the research question. This is consistent with the intention and appropriate methodological applications of the qualitative descriptive approach, which here provides a comprehensive summary, through the presentation of the facts relating to everyday events, as well as facilitation of the gathering of detailed descriptions of the factors affecting the dental practices of female dentists, of which there is little evidence in the literature to date (54). The methodology also requires that the researcher remain closer to the data and the surface of the words used to describe the concerns from the perspective of the participants, meaning that specific attention to relevant interpretations guided by the research question itself is essential (54).

The role of the researcher is to identify useful themes, select those that are most relevant to the study, and disclose them to the reader (56). In this manner, the study engages a fundamental qualitative approach in a description of a precise account of the concerns and issues that most participants would agree could affect their practice patterns, whereas the participants' role is to describe the factors that direct their dental practice. Therefore, their narratives are accepted as the construction of naturalism. As researchers, we describe their narratives to stakeholders. Thus, there are no facts outside of the particular context that gives them meaning, and the descriptions rely on the perceptions and sensibilities of the describer (54, 57–59). The spotlight is on direct communication with the research participants, recording their narratives, converting this into text, and writing accurate and detailed descriptions of the phenomena of interest. Our intention was to gain specific inside knowledge from female dentists to begin to better understand how each of the research participants experiences her world, individually and collectively.

The findings of our study potentially have the capacity to provide policy-makers, admissions personnel at dental schools, private dental business owners, and dental human resources professionals at hospitals with clear and usable information that can help them understand the characteristics of the particular healthcare providers we assessed. Sandelowski (2000) added that a qualitative descriptive approach is utilized when answers to the research question are of special relevance to practitioners (in our case, female dentists) and policy-makers (54).

4.2 Research Design

A researcher should select a design that favourably aligns with the topic and population of interest to answer the proposed research question (60). We accordingly decided to choose a qualitative descriptive research design with the intention of describing the issues that influence the practice profiles of female dentists. As Sandelowski (2000) claimed, a qualitative descriptive design is the methodology of choice when a researcher asks questions and seeks a straightforward and accurate description of a phenomenon (54). Furthermore, qualitative research helps the researcher to gain a description of human experiences, such as those of female dentists. Qualitative descriptive studies are a means of accurately describing what already exists, determining the frequency with which something occurs, and categorizing material to inform a specific topic of interest (61).

4.3 Participants

Within the frame of this study, we recruited a purposive sample of six female dentists, who are either general practitioners or specialists in the greater region of Montreal in Quebec, Canada. The participants were recruited from the dental clinics located in Montreal General Hospital. The associate dean of clinical affairs at the McGill faculty of dentistry introduced the researcher to a group of working female dentists. The research then contacted all participants via email to first request their participation. The sample size of six is sufficient to meet the rigours of an in-depth and detailed pilot study (62, 63). However, the sample, composed of general practitioners and specialists, was unbalanced because we were interviewing very busy people who gave up their time to share their experiences. We used particular inclusion and exclusion criteria.

Inclusion criteria:

- Female dentists who are general practitioners or specialists.

- At least 2 years of experience (to obtain the views of those most experienced in the field).

- 30 year old and over.

- English-speaking.

- Montreal residents.

Exclusion criteria:

- Under 2 years of experience (to ensure that the dentists included have acquired sufficient experience to have encountered the concerns that could influence their dental practice).

- Any dental care professionals other than female dentists (e.g., dental students, dental assistants).

4.4 Data Collection

Qualitative research relies on methods that permit researchers to delve into the attitudes, concerns, behaviours, and experiences of participants. The aim of our study meant that we conducted individual semi-structured interviews with open-ended questions to allow the participants to explain their views and concerns fully and in detail (64), recognizing that a set of closed questions may not permit the participants to express as much detailed information regarding their thoughts and beliefs. We used several key questions that acted as a guide to define certain areas that had to be explored; allowing the interviewer and interviewee to diverge from the topic to pursue an idea or response in more detail (65).

4.4.1 Interviews

Each participant was interviewed separately and privately in her private office or home. The interviews included several semi-structured open-ended questions, which was designed and used by the research team for the sole purpose of this study (Appendix I). The participants were encouraged to talk freely about their experiences.

The interviews lasted for approximately 60 to 90 minutes. However, the length and direction of each interview varied according to the participant's responses. The interviews were audio-recorded with the permission and written consent of the participants (Appendix II). Audio recording reduces the potential bias and misinterpretations that could result from a focus on the notes, rather than on the interviewee or the interviewer's memory. In addition, the recording assists in providing a detailed account of the participant's responses and a verbatim transcript for analysis.

4.5 Data Analysis

The rationale of the data analysis is to describe the participants' narrative accounts about a topic to answer the research question. Parahoo (2006) suggested that data analysis be conducted simultaneously and after completion of data collection (60).

Therefore, for the sake of coherence, the interviewer used qualitative content analysis to examine the data, which is the strategy of preference when conducting a qualitative descriptive study (51, 54). Hsieh and Shannon (2005) defined qualitative content analysis as a research method for the subjective interpretation of the content of text data through the systematic classification process of coding and identifying patterns (66). In contrast with quantitative content analysis, qualitative content analysis goes further than counting words, by examining data for contextual meanings, themes, and patterns (54). In addition, it allows the researcher to better understand the social and professional contextual reality of the text (67). The process of qualitative content analysis is divided into several systematic steps: preparing the data; defining the unit of analysis; developing categories and a coding scheme; coding the text; and producing the final report (67). We used data analysis software NVivo (version 9), which allows researchers to organize and sort their data, yielding maximum benefits by providing a systematic approach to data storage and handling (68).

We used the following steps suggested by Zhang and Wildemuth (2009) as follows:

Data Preparation

We began preparation by transcribing the interviews verbatim and comparing the written transcripts with the audio-recorded interviews to ensure accuracy. The transcripts were read and reread until we gained a holistic understanding of the interview content. Key words and phrases were highlighted and notes were taken.

Unit of Analysis

The transcribed interview was the first defined unit of analysis. We then summarized and analyzed each transcript in its entirety, and condensed the large data set into smaller units of text to permit further analysis.

Developing Categories and Coding Scheme

Coding was based on inductive and deductive processes. In inductive coding, coded categories emerged on the basis of the highlighted words and labels. Categories and minor categories were grouped on the basis of similarities and differences and the participants' own words as they appeared in the interview. This process went back and forth. The deductive coding originated from my own theoretical understandings (69).

Coding the Text

We carried out initial testing of the coding scheme by coding a sample text, and then checked and achieved coding consistency when we reached a final consensus. We used the same process to code the entire text, and we repeatedly assessed the coding consistency (70, 71).

Producing the Report

We reported the findings by describing the influences on the participants' dental practice in their own terms, using the themes that emerged from this study, which relate to the research questions.

4.6 Ethical Considerations

We obtained ethical approval to conduct the planned study from the Institutional Review Board of McGill University, after which we asked each participant to sign a consent form (Appendix II).

4.7 Trustworthiness

To support trustworthiness in this qualitative descriptive study, it was important to illustrate the richness of the data and convey it to the reader by an explicit representation of the congruence between the themes identified and the statements made by the participants (72). We used the following criteria to establish trustworthiness in this study.

4.7.1 Credibility

We hoped that the participants' view of the factors that might influence their practice was congruent with our reconstruction and representation of the same. We described extracts of the stories as closely as possible to the context and meaning attributed by the participants, so there is low inference (73). Furthermore, we ensured credibility by member checking by contacting the participants at the end of the study to confirm the findings (74).

4.7.2 Confirmability

Confirmability refers to the degree to which the results of a study can be confirmed or corroborated by others. We upheld this principle through an audit trail, which enabled the observer to go through the entire process of the research and the procedures described (75).

4.7.3 Transferability

Transferability refers to the ability of others to find meaning in the research findings in similar settings and contexts (72). It is the researcher's responsibility to present sufficient contextual information to the readers to allow them to establish such a transfer (55). In this study, the researcher checked her understanding of the participants' views with the participants themselves, as a form of member-checking.

5. FINDINGS

5.1 Description of the Participants

The participants consisted of two non-Canadian and four Canadian female dentists, whose ages ranged from 32 to 55 years, with a mean of 40.3 years. All but one of the six participants were married, and four had children living at home (Table 3).

Table 3. Percentage Distribution by Marital Status and Children Living at Home

Marital status	N
Single	1
Married	5
Total	6

Children living at home	4
Yes	2
No	6
Total	

Five of the participants were general practitioners, one was a specialist in orofacial pain, and one held a master's degree in dental science. The participants had 2 to 28 years of experience in dentistry, with approximately four reporting that they had at least 10 years' experience (Table 4). Four are currently working full-time, and the other two are working part-time. Those who reported working full-time explained that they had had to work part-time for some time, while on maternity leave, and mentioned being able to care for their child, including breast-feeding, as a significant consideration with regard to working part-time. Of the six participants, three indicated that they currently work 5 days per week, two reported working 4 days per week, and one indicated that she works 2 days per week. Only two of the participants own their practice; of the remaining four, one reported owning her practice for 4 years, before giving it up to have children. Five of the participants stated that they work in a group practice (Table 5). All six participants asserted that they selectively provide preventive management, operative treatments, simple endodontic and periodontal treatments, and implant restoration. None of the participants indicated that they provide surgical procedures or implant placements.

Table 4. Percentage Distribution by Professional Status and Year of Experience	
Professional status	N
General Practitioner	5
Specialists	1
Total	6
Years of experience	
0-9	2
10-20	3
20-30	1
Total	6

Table 5. Percentage Distribution by Practice Characteristics

Working full-time or part-time	N
Full-time	4
Part-time	2
Total	6

Working days per week	
2 days	1
4 days	2
5 days	3
Total	6

Working solo or in a group practice	
Solo practice	1
Group practice	5
Total	6

Practice ownership	
Yes	2
No	4
Total	6

5.2 Appraising the Research Question

With regard to answering our proposed research question, the analysis yielded five major categories related to the issues that influenced the decision-making of female dentists regarding their practice. These were (a) family responsibilities, (b) workplace settings, (c) societal/family obligations, (d) economics, and (e) individual preference.

5.2.1 Family Responsibilities

"Balance is not better time management, but better boundary management. Balance means making choices and enjoying those choices"

Betsy Jacobson (76)

The six participants provided insight into their personal and professional lives, and discussed the issues, related to family expectations and perspectives, which have influenced their dental practice patterns. A significant focus of returning to family responsibilities dominated the topic of choice of these women throughout the interviews. Family responsibilities included marriage, caring for children, and other household activities.

Female dentists' decisions regarding their practice profile also appear to be guided by another family matter; marriage. They apparently tend to make costly choices regarding their practice once they plan to get married. One participant declared that she had to quit her private practice because she got married and wanted to have a family and children, and she decided to keep working as an associate because it would enable her to both work and have children at the same time.

Well, that's when I made a choice. When I met my husband and we were going to get married, I gave up my private practice because I was in a partnership, and I had bought into a partnership that wasn't very advantageous to me, so when the time came, I could make a decision of either staying and working harder—you know to build up my practice to a better level—or just give it up, and go back to working as an associate.

It is difficult for female dentists to pursue their professional careers and simultaneously be fulfilled as wives and as successful mothers. One participant stated that she did not want to concentrate on any dental specialty, and preferred to practice as a general practitioner, because she was married and wanted to have a family:

Because I got married one year after I graduated, after my residency—and by the time you graduate, you are almost 30 years old, so you better start a family, so you start having kids.

Female dentists appear to view themselves as the second earners in their families, and they tend not to engage themselves in hectic life stressors. This is in contrast with their male counterparts, who will place clearly defined boundaries between their family responsibilities and their professional lives, as they are perceived as the main wage earners in their families.

You should manage your life and everything, but comparing to men…because you know they are not that involved with the kids and everything, so you have to manage between your life, the kids, and then the work.

According to this participant, female dentists bear a larger share of family demands than do male dentists. Moreover, female dentists who are married to a partner with a highly demanding job will juggle family and work duties more. Our study participants, as female dentists, take on the challenge of being everything to everyone, and these expectations are accepted as having to be met on a daily basis. According to one participant, who is married to a man who works long hours, she has no choice but to reduce her working hours, and one stated that it is her duty to take care of the house, along with her professional issues, because her husband's job is so demanding. The following sentiment echoes this:

> *I can see like some day that can be a problem, because my husband's job is so demanding, it is really my responsibility to make sure that the house and all of our professional things, like our insurance, our disability insurance, everything is taking care of right, so all the banking, the accountants, the lawyers—all of that has to be taken care of by me, which means working five days a week would be a struggle.*

It was made clear that a good family-work balance is an important goal; otherwise, these constant conflicts may lead to additional stresses. It can be expected that the life-work balance becomes easier to attain when the workplace helps female dentists to achieve their family goals and participate in family activities, while simultaneously facilitating success in their trained profession.

5.2.1.1 Childcare Responsibilities

The participants associated their role as mother with childcare responsibilities, which included discussions about maternity leave, breast-feeding, and taking care of their children. Four stated that they had needed to take maternity leave for a couple of months to take care of their newborns, while one participant reported that, even after maternity leave, she had to work part-time for 9 months in order to continue breast-feeding:

I took about six months off for each of the kids. When I came back for three months.....back full-time after nine months for each of them. I was still breast-feeding and so I wanted to still be.

Another participant explained that it was difficult for her to manage work and having children at the same time, explaining that she had had to reassess her life priorities at the beginning. She consequently decided to build her private practice first, which had its own challenges that were made more difficult by the fact that she had to take maternity leave for a few months, which was disruptive to her practice:

It was not easy at the beginning, but you have to set priorities, so at the beginning, I had my practice; I did a residency until '85, and I opened my private practice with somebody else. And it's not easy because, at the beginning, you have to stop sometimes for maternity leave.

She further explained that she had worked on a part-time basis until her second child was born, and then started working full-time when this child turned a year old. However, she declared that working full-time was a struggle, as she had to manage work and home activities simultaneously:

For sure, I had to work part-time for a little while until the second child was born. Only when the child was born and maybe one year old, then you can start to go full-time. Full-time is still hard because you have to juggle work and home.

The tension created by trying to balance work and childcare responsibilities affects female dentists because they believe it is a woman's place to raise her children. Consider the stress of a full-time job and the added responsibilities for women dentists to deal with high-stress work and the demands of childcare obligations. The quotes above allow us to begin to understand that returning to work after maternity leave may present significant challenges for many female dentists. Our participants appeared to feel stressed around the extra tension created by their own perspectives, responsibilities, and expectations, with regard to maintaining their professional lives and devoting themselves to full-time motherhood. They also seemed to feel anxious about returning to their professional life after giving birth, and reluctant to leave their children.

One participant asserted that she has never worked full-time since she had her three children, and she now only works 2 to 3 days a week. She stated that she prefers to work part-time because she is very busy raising her children, and this arrangement became a suitable way for her to manage working and taking care of her children concurrently:

> That's why I don't work full-time because I am really busy with them...you know...I just work part-time and the rest ...spend time with them and, yeah, take care of them.

Many female dentists find it difficult to manage their professional lives and maintain their roles as mothers. Childcare obligations are difficult to combine with a full-time job that comes with the expectations of a high workload. Thus, it is important that they overcome their daily struggle to balance work and family. The following quote is from one participant who decided not to embark on her professional journey as a landlord dentist, and to have children instead:

> I was trying to figure out whether or not I should really venture out on my own or if I should stay an associate. Then I figured that it would be better to

stay an associate while I wanted to have kids so that it wouldn't be so stressful.

Having children may greatly affect female dentists' decision-making regarding their professional future. Given the stress involved, many may sacrifice their careers to have children. It is very difficult to combine childcare responsibilities with work; the balance is jeopardized because the demands to do both and to do them well are extremely challenging. Our participants felt more obliged to take care of their children than their partners, in line with socially accepted perceptions regarding gender roles within the family unit. One participant indicated that she chose to leave her private practice and to raise her children instead:

It was very hard; it took a long time for me to accept that. I had to make a decision, so I had to make a choice and between choosing to have a family and kids and maintaining a private practice; I chose my kids.

The pursuit of a balance between work and family appeared to be difficult to maintain, suggesting that we must make this more explicit and open to discussion. This further suggests that there should be greater flexibility to allow female dentists to negotiate their priorities across their work and their children. Although our participants have been striving to achieve the goal of a balanced life, they tend to have the luxury of choosing to be a mother, rather than a practicing dentist. This suggests that being a dentist is only a way for them to provide financial support for their children and families. One participant said:

If you ask me which is the priority?, I would say, being a mother is the priority and that being a dentist is really just a means for providing for my kids. It's not to say that I don't love dentistry. I do love what I'm doing, but in the grand scheme of things, it's a way for me to provide for my kids, my family.

Having both children and a bright future remained a concern for the newly married dentist in our study, who admitted that while she would love to continue working on a full-time basis, she was concerned that her enthusiasm for her work might change after having children:

Well, to me, I think it is because of family. I am young, I am newly married, but I don't have children yet, so I like to work, and I am a worker bee, so I think I will work full-time. I would like to continue to work full-time forever, for the rest of my career. I say this now, but I don't have children right that is different.

According to Walton et al. (2004), when family and work obligations clash, female dentists are far more likely than their male counterparts to cut back on their working hours. They found that having children reduces women's work hours by an average of nearly 1 day per week (30). One participant said:

I think, as a female dentist, it seems more reasonable to stay home because the kid has ped day right.

"The good news is superwoman is dead. The bad news is she left behind an entire generation of women who are still struggling to figure out how to balance home and work." Marian Thomas (77)

5.2.2 Workplace Settings

Another major category arising from the iterative process of content analysis concerned the workplace setting. The participants mentioned issues related to their work settings that played a role in their practice. The context of the workplace environment falls into three minor categories: the nature of the workplace, insecure working conditions, and negative experiences with partners.

5.2.2.1 Nature of the workplace

The professional practice of many female dentists appears to be determined by the characteristics of the dental office in which they work. Every dental office has its own practice standards, protocols, and culture, and both dental offices and hospitals should meet appropriate and high standards of dental care to ensure the recruitment of a large number of highly qualified dental care professionals. However, one participant said:

While I was looking for my second and third part-time positions, I mean without leaving the first one, because I did finally find other clinics that were more organised, that were better in following the protocols for infection control and treatment protocols for various types of dentistry.

The context of the workplace setting is a powerful tool in attracting female dental professionals and encouraging them to perform more effectively. Following standards and protocols is important, not only to attract a greater number of professionals, but also to prevent harmful dentistry.

I found it very disappointing because you think that once you get out of university that you are going to be heading toward this nice clinic that follows protocols that you have learned through dental school in terms of

sterilisation, management of cases, [and] dental treatment standards, and
sometimes I saw things at that office that I found a little bit unnerving.

This participant's description of her experience practicing dentistry in a private dental clinic supports the aforementioned claim that workplace strategy influences the practice profile of female dentists. She mentioned that the dental clinic where she worked did not meet her expectations of dental care. Dental offices must be established with a primary goal of meeting the needs of female dentists, to support and improve their performance if they mean to retain this cohort of professionals.

5.2.2.2 Insecure working conditions

There is apparently a relationship between work conditions and the performance of female dentists. An insecure work environment appears to provide these professionals with fascinating challenges and concerns regarding their future. An insecure work environment might force female dentists to become dissatisfied and start looking for other places to work. One participant recounted her concerns by saying:

With everything that's happening with the MUHC ..... now, my future was
not so clear as far as where I would be able to practice, and so I felt now is
a good time to at least take a step out the door to secure something for
myself and [my] future.

This participant felt insecure and uncertain, yet she decided to move her practice from the hospital setting to another private clinic in order to protect her future. In addition, insecure working conditions seemed to affect our participants' job satisfaction, interfere with their performance, and disrupt their career options.

5.2.2.3 Negative Experience with Partners

One participant gave an account of an unpleasant experience with her partner that negatively affected her private practice and influenced her decision to sacrifice it. The following quote justifies her choice:

Well, like I said, I had to sacrifice because I had a bad partner. If I didn't have a bad partnership, if those three to four years that I had my practice…if my partner had helped me build it up to the point where it was running very smoothly, I would have kept the practice and I would have had my kids, because then you would have somebody there supporting you.

A collaborative relationship appears to be important to ensure the sharing of best practices and to provide high-quality care to patients. Effective teamwork is necessary for the success of any dental practice, and more so for female dentists. The failure to implement effective teamwork and inter-professional collaborative relationships might result in unintentional harm to patients.

5.2.3 Societal Obligation

Social perspectives of responsibilities have also been identified as issues that could influence the career decisions and preferences of female dentists. Unlike those who are married, who are likely to make their schedules more family-friendly, unmarried female dentists tend to seek work that suits their needs and social/family commitments.

I picked a private practice that suited my schedule and my needs. One of the things I didn't want…I didn't want to work weekends and minimal evenings. I just like having my evenings free for me for my social life.

Female dentists face multiple societal obligations. Given their chosen profession, they must find ways of reconciling their professional demands with their perceived personal obligations, which relate to their friends and themselves. However, they may rise to the task; these women can be dentists, while simultaneously being friends, mothers, sisters, daughters, or wives. It is all a matter of choosing a line of work that fits their social obligations and way of life.

5.2.4 Economics

I was looking for another job because, when I graduated in '94 and in '95 after the residency program, in Montreal, the economy was not that great, so I had to find eventually three part-time positions to have a full-time job.

It has become apparent that economics affects medical practice profiles in all professions. In turn, economics is also affected by each individual's practice profile. Being a health-related service, dentistry is subject to the highly volatile economic cycles that affect all sectors of society. For example, during times in which interest rates are high, female dentists will be more inclined to work a greater number of days per week and on a full-time basis. This will allow them to earn more money, save more, and generate more income, via increased interest. One of our study participants further noted:

It was a very difficult time because it was 1984, when there was a lot of unemployment, and the interest rate was 18%, so it was very hard to set up a practice, so then I did a one-year residency, and then I got into an associateship for one year, and then after that, I opened the office with somebody else, with a partner, but the interest rate was very high. So it was very hard for at least five years.

Conversely, during strained economic times, such as those experienced in 2009, during the height of the world's latest economic recession, dentists' net incomes decreased by more than 5% (78). Such a decline in income will naturally affect how a dentist manages their practice; renewing depreciated equipment, maintaining modern installations, and investing in educated and experienced staff requires capital.

5.2.5 Individual Preference

One final consideration is related to the individual preferences of female dentists. Naturally, each practice profile will be different, because all individuals are different. A dentist's practice is directly affected by needs, wants, preferences, and ideals. If a female dentist is to be successful in her practice, it must be set up in a manner that is consistent with who she is and what she wants.

Because I have a lot to do—you know, the other days I have other stuff to do—and I like it that way.

6. DISCUSSION

My interviews with the six female dentists who participated in this study revealed that family responsibilities, workplace settings, societal obligation, economics, and individual preference are all interwoven into their practice profiles. However, the majority of our participants were concerned with family responsibilities, so we concluded that the latter have the greatest impact on the practices of female dentists. This is consistent with the results of a study conducted by Naidoo, which identified a woman's dual responsibility at home and at work as being a major factor influencing the work patterns of female dentists in South Africa (79). These healthcare providers are more likely than their male counterparts to take on domestic responsibilities within households when they start a family (34, 80, 81).

An additional source of motivation for female dentists, who choose their career for independence, self-employment, and altruistic purposes, is earning income. However, these women's careers are often interrupted by the demands of their family and childcare responsibilities (13, 80), so they must spend a great deal of time away from their job. Female dentists who have children are expected to cope with the responsibility of dedicated childcare. They are constantly trying to negotiate a balance between these two life domains to ensure that their productivity is not affected. Furthermore, failure to directly address the tension between professional and family life may cause adverse consequences, such as stress and burnout syndrome (82). It has been suggested that one method of promoting the quality of a work environment that favours female dentists is to encourage the use of frameworks and standards in developing "family-friendly" workplaces, which requires concrete policy approaches (83). An example of this is the use of standards for childcare provision at the national level to promote a balance between work life and family life (84). Another specific element includes maternity-related issues, whereby the work environment policies must consider pregnancy as a natural event and provide arrangements that accommodate the needs of pregnant women (85). These approaches necessitate action from national policies and regulatory bodies, but will incentivize female dental practitioners to better balance the demands of their work and family lives.

Our study participants identified workplace settings, environment, and culture as some of the elements that influence their practice choices. The workplace setting positively influences the practice choices of female dentists; they perform better when working conditions are adjusted to accommodate their specific needs during certain transitional stages (i.e., marriage/family) of their lives and careers. Female dentists need a professional working space, and they must have the capacity to set limits and determine acceptable behaviours at their places of work in order to be comfortable, professional, and feel included. Similar findings were observed in a South African study, in which poor working conditions were highly associated with job dissatisfaction (86). Bodur (2001) investigated rationales for job satisfaction levels in healthcare staff employed at health centers in Turkey. The results showed that low levels of job satisfaction were primarily due to substandard working conditions (87). A study assessing levels of nurses' job satisfaction revealed that employees who were content with their working conditions tended to be more productive and committed to their jobs (88). Female dentists may choose not to practice to their fullest potential when they are dissatisfied with their working conditions, including their associates/partners at work. Ayers (2005) suggested that the working environment should motivate employees to perform at their best and show commitment to the organization, improving working conditions to support the organization's mission, thereby impacting on job satisfaction and work effectiveness (89). The conditions under which work is performed can have a substantial impact on people's effectiveness and comfort. Indeed, working conditions should meet the values and aspirations of female dentists and all other healthcare providers.

Societal obligation may also influence female dentists' practice choices. Many of the challenges that face unmarried female dentists appear to be based on social attitudes. In many cases, if these professional single women were to give sufficient time to their careers, it would mean sacrificing their social lives. In this manner, we can say that female dentists experience hardship from the influence of social obligation and societal restriction. Risser et al. (1996) identified the time commitment and social compromises as the principal deterrents to entering the field of oral and maxillofacial surgery among female dental students in the United States (90). Female dentists entering the workplace today are at the vanguard of advanced technology that, in the near future, will make the performance of dentistry especially stimulating and satisfying. Female dentists are recognized as being proficient, reliable, civic-minded individuals, but societal obligations appear to obstruct their achievement and success in their chosen career (90).

Our participants also raised the issues of economics and financial matters; a female dentist may execute her career in dentistry within the standards of fulfilling her economic needs, and may develop the proficiency and clinical capability for independent broad practice, consisting of knowledge of health advancement and related obstacles. Fulfillment of economic requirements, particularly for female dentists, is an important element in the process of appraisal and evaluation of the types of the practices they perform. Through her profession, a female dentist can easily support her family. Working longer hours becomes even more of a necessity should the high interest rate scenario arise and the female dentist has, for example, house or car loans to repay. Facing monetary issues such as these, female dentists would prefer to work in high-salaried positions, rather than work in positions with a lower salary and have to supplement their income by working extra hours.

Decisions regarding what, where, when, and how to practice are influenced by numerous factors, including personal preferences (91). Personal preference has also been identified as a key factor in helping to influence career choices and workforce participation of doctors in their postgraduate years in Australia (92). Female dentists may choose to practice part-time or only a few days a week as an individual choice, or they might decide to work part-time for various reasons, for example, to have free time in order to study or to simply to enjoy family life. They may decide to return to practice full-time when their children have grown older and are more independent, or when further education has been completed. Working full-time will bring focus to their careers and developmental growth. The crucial point is that female dentists should have the capacity to work when they are willing and able to do so.

7. CONCLUSION

We are witnessing a significant increase in the number of women choosing dentistry as a profession (93), which correlates with the number of women who are applying to dental schools (94). However, such changes provide new challenges and consequently necessitate an in-depth analysis and examination of the particular concerns and needs for women at work. Could this be an artefact of the traditional model of the male-oriented dental curriculum at schools?

A safe and secure working environment is fundamental to ensuring the effectiveness of the female dentist workforce. In this respect, a supportive working environment helps encouraging women to utilise their skills and knowledge to the best of their ability.

Women generally face a greater number of obstacles in order to succeed at work, and female dentists are no exception. The societal norm that suggests the primary role of women is to fulfill family responsibilities may be to blame. A well-designed, person-centred, education may fulfill the needs and roles of female dentists and better accommodate their life experiences. We suggest, that much of the tension experienced by female dentists, can be reduced by making explicit their concerns, challenges, and needs, in order to inform the ways in which we educate and describe professional practice.

8. REFERENCES

1. Adams TL. Feminization of professions: The case of women in dentistry. *Can J Sociol* 2005; 30:71–94.

2. Aguila MA, Leggott PJ, Robertson PB, Porterfield DL, Felber GD. Practice pattern among male and female general dentists in a Washington state population. *Am Dent Assoc* 2005;136:790–6.

3. Brennan DS, Spencer AJ, Szuster FS. Differences in time devoted to practice by male and female dentists. *Br Dent J* 1992;172:348–9.

4. Williams AP, Domnick-Pierre K, Vayada E, Stevenson HM, Burke M. Women in medicine: practice patterns and attitudes. *Can Med Assoc* 1990;143(3):194–201.

5. Williams PA. Changing the palace guard: analyzing the impact of women's entry into medicine. *Gend Work Organ* 1999;6(2):106–21.

6. Adams TL. Gender and feminization in health care professions. *Sociology Compass* 2010;4(7):454–465.

7. Reskin B, Roos PA. Job queues, gender queues: *Explaining women's inroads into male occupations*. Philadelphia (PA): Temple University Press; 1990.

8. Boulis AK, Jacobs JA. *The changing face of medicine*. Ithaca (NY): ILR Press; 2008.

9. Elston MA. *Women and medicine: The future*. London UK: Royal College of Physicians; 2009.

10. Collin J. Les femmes dans la profession pharmaceutique au Quebec: rupture ou continuite? *Rech Femin* 1992;5(2):31–56.

11. Lindsay S. The feminization of the physician assistant profession. *Women Health* 2005;41:37–61.

12. Kaldenberg DO, Becker BW, Zvonkovic A. Work and commitment among young professionals: A study of male and female dentists. *Hum Relat* 1995;48(11):1355–1377.

13. Ayers KM, Thomson WM, Rich AM, Newton JT. Gender differences in dentists' working practices and job satisfaction. *J Dent* 2008;36(5):343–50.

14. Katrova LG. Gender impact on the socioprofessional identification of women dentists in Bulgaria. *J Dent Educ* 2004;68(7):19–22.

15. Gjerberg E. Gender similarities in doctors' preferences—and gender differences in final specializations. *Soc Sci Med* 2002;54:591–605.

16. Cassel J. Doing gender, doing surgery: Women surgeons in a man's profession. *Human Organization* 1997;56:47–52.

17. Hinze S. Gender and the body of medicine or at least some body parts: reconstructing the prestige hierarchy of medical specialties. *The Sociological Quarterly*1999;40:217–239.

18. Pringle R. *Sex and medicine: Gender, power and authority in the medical profession.* Cambridge (UK): Cambridge University Press; 1998.

19. Dominik G, Schäfe G. "Feminization" in German dentistry. Career paths and opportunities—a gender comparison. *Women's Studies International Forum* 2011;34:130–9.

20. Kuhlmann E. Gender differences, gender hierarchies and professions: an embedded approach to the German dental profession. *International Journal of Sociology and Social Policy* 2003;23(4/5):80–96.

21. Atchison KA, Bibb CA, Lefever KH, Mito RS, Lin S, Engelhardt R. Gender differences in career and practice patterns of PGD-trained dentists. *J Dent Edu* 2002;66(12):1358–1367.

22. Newton JT, Thorogood N, Gibbons DE. The work patterns of male and female dental practitioners in the United Kingdom. *Int Dent J* 2000;50:61–8.

23. Clark P, Martinez H, Ryan G, Barile L. Does being a woman make a difference in professional practice? A qualitative view to the practice of rheumatology. *J Rheumatol* 2000;27:2010–7.

24. Zillen PA, Mindak M. World dental demographics. *Int Dent J* 2000;50:194–7.

25. Widstrom E, Eaton KA, Borutta A, Dybizbaska E, Broukal Z. Oral healthcare in transition in Eastern Europe. *Br Dent J* 2001;190(11):580–4.

26. Perret, JB. La feminization dans la medicine dentaire. *Revue mensuelles iussed'odontostomatologie* 1990;100(10):1238–9.

27. Gonzalez Ortiz RM, Diaz de Kuri M. Women in dentistry. *J Hist Dent* 2001;49(1):37–41.

28. Niessen LC, Kleinman DV, Wilson AA. Practice characteristics of women dentists. *J Am Dent Assoc* 1986;113:883–8.

29. Spencer AJ, Lewis JM. The practice of dentistry by male and female dentists. *Community Dent Oral Epidemiol* 1998;16(4):202–207.

30. Walton SM, Byck GR, Cooksey JA, Kaste LM. Assessing differences in hours worked between male and female dentists: An analysis of cross-sectional national survey data from 1979 through 1999. *J Am Den Assoc* 2004;135(5):637–645.

31. Matthew RW, Scully C. Working patterns of male and female dentists in the UK. *Br Dent J* 1994;176(12):463–466.

32. Murray JJ. Better opportunities for women dentists: A review of the contribution of women dentists to the workforce. *Br Dent J* 2002;192:191–196.

33. Price SS. A profile of women dentists. *J Am Dent Assoc* 1990;120:403–8.

34. De Wet E, Truter M, Ligthelm AJ. Working patterns of male and female dentists in South Africa. *J Dent Assoc S Afr* 1997;52:15–7.

35.   Seward MH, McEwen ME. The provision of dental care by women dentists in England and Wales in 1985: A 10 year review. *Br Dent J* 1987;162(2):50–1.

36.   Dolan TA. Gender trends in dental practice patterns. A review of current U.S. literature. *J Am Coll Dent* 1991;58(3):12–8.

37.   Newton JT, Thorogood N, Gibbons DE. A study of the career development of male and female dental practitioners. *Br Dent J* 2000;188:90–94.

38.   Brown LJ, Lazar V. Differences in net incomes of male and female owner general practitioners. *J Am Dent Assoc* 1998;129(3):373–8.

39.   American Dental Association. 1995 survey of dentists. *A comparison of male and female dentists: Work-related issues.* Chicago, IL:ADA, 1997.

40.   Muzzin LJ, Brown GP, Hornosty RW. Consequences of feminization of a profession: the case of Canadian pharmacy. *Women and Health* 1994;21:39–56.

41.   Pew Research Center. (January 19 2010). *New economics of marriage: the rise of wives*. January 19, 2010. Available at http://pewresearch.org/pubs/1466/economics-marriage-rise-of-wives.

42.   Glimour J, Stewardson DA, Shugars DA, Burke FJ. An assessment of career satisfaction among a group of general dental practitioners in Staffordshire. *Br Dent J* 2005;198:701–4.

43.   Luzzi L, Spencer AJ, Jones K, Teusner D. Job satisfaction of registered dental practitioners. *Aust Dent J* 2005;50(3):179–185.

44.   Cooper C, Watts J, Kelly M. Job satisfaction, mental health and job stressors among general dental practitioners in the UK. *Br Dent J* 1987;162:77–81.

45.   Cooper C, Watts J, Baglioni AJ Jr, Kelly M. Occupational stress amongst general practice dentists. *J Occup Psychol* 1988;61:163–74.

46.   Humphris GM, Peacock L. Occupational stress and job satisfaction in the community dental service of north Wales: A pilot study. *Community Dent Health* 1992;10:73–82.

47. Harris RV, Ashcroft A, Burnside G, Dancer JM, Smith D, Grieveson B. Facets of job satisfaction of dental practitioners working in different organizational settings in England. *Br Dent J* 2008;204:E1; discussion 16–17.

48. Harris R, Burnside G, Ashcroft A, Grieveson B. Job satisfaction of dental practitioners before and after a change in incentives and governance: a longitudinal study. *Br Dent J* 2009;207:E4-E5.

49. Shugars DA, DiMatteo RM, Hats RD, Cretin S, Johnson JD. Professional satisfaction among California general dentists. *J Dent Educ* 1990;54:661–669.

50. Wells A, Winter PA. Influence of practice and personal characteristics on dental job satisfaction. *J Dent Educ* 1999;63:805–812.

51. Neergaard MA, Olesen F, Andersen RS, Sondergaard J. Qualitative description——the poor cousin of health research? *BMC Med Res Methodol* 2009;9:52.

52. Milne J, Oberle K. Enhancing rigor in qualitative description. *Journal of Wound, Ostomy & Continence Nursing* 2005;32(6):413–20.

53. Sullivan-Bolyai S, Bova C, Harper D. Developing and refining interventions in persons with health disparities: the use of qualitative description. *Nursing Outlook* 2005;53:127–33.

54. Sandelowski M. Focus on research methods: Whatever happened to qualitative description? *Res Nurs & Health* 2000;23 (4):334–40.

55. Lincoln YS, Guba EG. *Naturalistic inquiry*. Beverly Hills (CA): Sage; 1985.

56. Braun V, Clarke V. Using thematic analysis in psychology. *Qualitative Research in Psychology* 2006;3:77–101.

57. Emerson RM, Fretz RI, Shaw LL. *Writing ethnographic field notes*. Chicago (IL): University of Chicago Press; 1995.

58. Giorgi A. Description versus interpretation: competing alternative strategies for qualitative research. *J Phenomenol Psychol* 1992;23:119–35.

59. Wolcott HF. *Transforming qualitative data: description, analysis & interpretation.* Thousand Oaks, CA: Saga; 1994.

60. Parahoo K. *Nursing research: Principles, process and issues* (2nd ed). Basingstoke, England: Palgrave Macmillan; 2006.

61. Marriner A. *Research design: survey/descriptive. Readings for nursing research.* St. Louis: Mosby; 1981.

62. Miles MB, Huberman AM. *Qualitative data analysis: an expanded sourcebook* (2nd ed). Thousand Oaks, CA: Sage; 1994.

63. Patton M. *Qualitative evaluation and research methods.* London: Sage; 1990.

64. Mason J. *Qualitative researching.* London (UK): Sage; 1996.

65. Britten N. Qualitative interviews in medical research. *BMJ* 1995;311:251–3.

66. Hsieh HF, Shannon SE. Three approaches to qualitative content analysis. *Qual Health Res* 2005;15 (9):1277–1288.

67. Zhang Y, Wildemuth B. Qualitative analysis of content. In Wildemuth B, editor. *Applications of social research methods to questions in information and library services.* Westport (CT): Libraries Unlimited; 2009: pp. 308–19.

68. Davies MB. *Doing a successful research project: using qualitative or quantitative methods.* Houndmills: Palgrave MacMillan; 2007.

69. Elo S, Kyngas H. The qualitative content analysis process. *J Adv Nurs* 2008;62(1):107–15.

70. Weber RP. *Basic content analysis.* Newbury Park, CA: Sage Publications; 1990.

71. Zhang Y, Wildemuth BM. Qualitative analysis of content. In *Applications of social research methods to questions in information and library science edn.*

Edited by Wildemuth B. Santa Barbara, CA: Greenwood Press; 2009:308–319.

72.   LioBiondo-Wood, G, Haber J. *Nursing research: Methods and critical appraisal for evidence-based practice* (6th ed). St Louis, MO: Mosby; 2006.

73.   Tobin GA, Begley CM. Methodological rigour within a qualitative framework. *J Adv Nurs* 2004;48(4):388–96.

74.   Polit DF, Beck CT. *Essentials of nursing research: appraising evidence for nursing practice* (7th ed). Philadelphia: Wolters Kluwer Health, Lippincott Williams & Wilkins, Philadelphia; 2010.

75.   Shenton AK. Strategies for ensuring trustworthiness in qualitative research projects. *Educ Inform* 2004;22:63–75.

76.   Jacobson B. (2011), Quotation by Betsy Jacobson. Available from: http://www.yourlifebalancecoach.com/blog/2011/06/favorite-life-balance-quotes/ (Accessed 13 May 2013)

77.   Thomas M. *Balancing career and family: Overcoming the superwoman syndrome*. Shawnee Mission, KS: National Press Publications; 1990.

78.   Pollock S. *Economic factors affect dental trends*. Available from: http://blog.go-iba.org/index.php/2010/05/21/economic-factors-affect-dental-trends/

79.   Naidoo S. Women in dentistry in South Africa: A survey of their experiences and opinions. *J Dent Assoc S Afr* 2005;60(7):284, 6, 8.

80.   Ashri NY, Norah Al Ajaji, Mayyadah Al Mozainy, Rasha Al Sourani. Career profile of dentists in Saudi Arabia. *Saudi Dent J* 2009;21:28–36.

81.   Smith MK, Dundes L. The implications of gender stereotypes for the dentist-patient relationship. *J Dent Educ* 2008;72(5):562–70.

82. Hansen N, Sverke M, Naswall K. Predicting nurse burnout from demands and resources in three acute care hospitals under different forms of ownership: a cross-sectional questionnaire survey. *Int J Nurs Stud* 2009;46(1),96–107.

83. Voss E. Working conditions and social dialogue—national frameworks, empirical findings and experience of good practice at enterprise level in six European countries (Draft Report). *European Foundation for the Improvement of Living and Working Conditions; 2009.* Available from: http://www.eurofound.europa.eu/docs/events/confworkcond09/draftreport.p df (Accessed 10 April 2010)

84. Council of the European Union. Guidelines for the employment policies of the Member States (integrated guidelines 17–24). In: Council Decision on guidelines for the employment policies of the Member States. Legislative Acts and other Instruments (10614/2/08 REV 2). *Brussels: Council of the European Union; 2008.*Available from: http:// register.consilium.europa.eu/pdf/en/08/st10/st106 14-re02.en08.pdf (Accessed 2 Jul 2010)

85. Wisckow C, Albreht T, de Pietro C. How to create an attractive and supportive working environment for health professionals. *Health Systems and Policy Analysis 2010.* Available from: http://www.euro.who.int/_data/assests/pdf_file/0018/124416/e94293.pdf

86. Kekana HP, Du Rand EA, VanWyk NC. Job satisfaction of registered nurses in a community hospital in the Limpopo Province in South Africa. *Curationis* 2007;30(2):24–35.

87. Bodur S. Job satisfaction of healthcare staff employed at health centers in Turkey. *Occup Med* (Lond). 2002;52(6):353–5.

88. Al-Hussami M. A study of nurses' job satisfaction: the relationship to organizational commitment, perceived organizational support, transactional leadership, transformational leadership and level of education. *Eur J Sci Res* 2008;22(2):286–295.

89. Ayers, K. Creating a responsible workplace. *Human Resources Magazine 2005*.Available from:
http://findarticles.com/p/articles/mi_m3495/is_2_50/ai_n11841926

90. Risser MJ, Laskin DM. Women in oral and maxillofacial surgery: factors affecting career choices, attitudes and practice characteristics. *J Oralmaxillofac Surg* 1996;54(6):753–7.

91. The physician workforce: projections and research into current issues affecting supply and demand. *U.S. department of health and human services health resources and services administration bureau of health professions.* December 2008.

92. Australian Medical Advisory Committee, Career decision making by doctors in their postgraduate years: A Literature Review. *AMWAC Report 2002.1,* February 2002. AMWAC: Sydney, Australia.

93. Jeanne C. Sinkford. Global health through women's leadership: Introduction to the conference proceedings. *J Dent Educ* 2006;70:5–7.

94. Scarbecz M, Ross JA. Gender differences in first-year dental students' motivation to attend dental school. *J Dent Educ* 2002;66(8):952–61.

9. Appendix I

Interview Guide

Introduction

1. Please can you introduce yourself?
2. Would you elaborate further on your educational background?
3. Why did you choose to be a dentist?
4. What were your thoughts on dentistry?

Experience

5. Tell me about your experience in the dental school you attended.
6. Tell me about your experience of being a practicing female dentist.
7. Share with me any challenges you have faced throughout your career so far.
8. Describe to me your perceived feelings toward your work.

Current practice

9. Do you work in a private or public sector? Why?
10. Do you work full- time or part-time? Why?
11. How many hours do you work per week? Why?
12. How many patients do you see per day? Why?
13. Do you prefer to work in a group or a solo practice? Why?
14. Are you satisfied with your current practice? Why?
15. Share with me any barriers and motivators that you think could influence your practice.

10. Appendix II

Consent Form

Project title: Female dentists; their professional lives and concerns

Principle Investigator:
Shahrokh Esfandiari
Faculty of Dentistry
Oral Health and Society Division
3550 University Street, Rm 206
Montreal, Quebec H3A 2A7

Purpose of the Study:
To understand the factors that may affect decisions made by female dentists with regard to their practice.

Description/participation
Your participation in this study will be through an open conversation-style interview for a period of 60-90 minutes, and will be recorded for further analysis. Your name and affiliation will not be disclosed to anyone other than the interviewer. It is understood that your participation in this study is entirely voluntary, and you may choose not to participate or withdraw at any point before, during or after the interview. You are free to not answer specific questions during the interview, or to ask that any part of the interview not be recorded.

Potential Risks and Benefits:
No anticipated risks are associated with your participation in this study. The only cost to you will be the time needed for your collaboration. There will be no financial compensation for your participation in this study.

Confidentiality
The recorded interview will be handled with the utmost confidentiality. Your name and location will be concealed at all times and will never be published.

Contact:
If you have any further questions/concerns about this study please contact:
Shahrokh Esfandairi
Faculty of Dentistry
Oral Health and Society Division
3550 University Street
Montreal, Quebec H3A 2A7

_____   _____   ____ /_____ /___
Signature of Participant   Name (Printed)   day/month/year

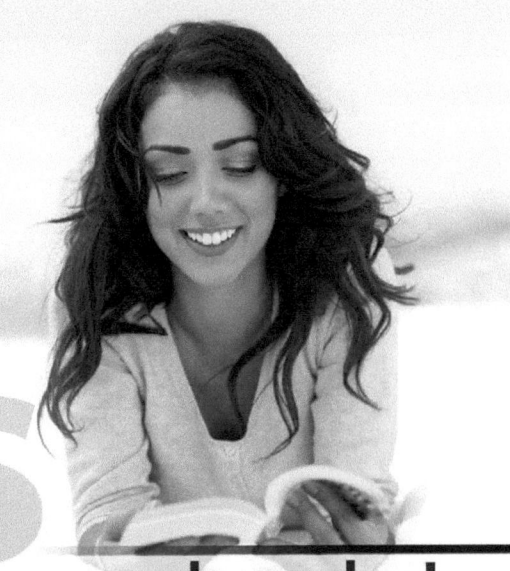
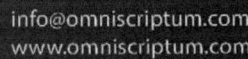 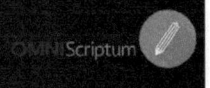

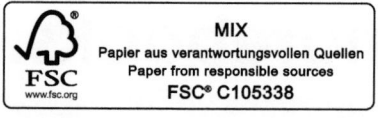

Printed by Books on Demand GmbH, Norderstedt / Germany